Silent Storm:
Inside the World of Asthma

What No One Tells You About Living, Breathing and Thriving with the World's Most Common Lung Disease

AF720000

Wachyudi Muchsin

Silent Storm: Inside the World of Asthma

What No One Tells You About Living, Breathing and Thriving with the World's Most Common Lung Disease

ELIVA PRESS

ISBN: 978-99993-4-406-7

Cover Design: Eliva Press
Cover Image: www.ingimage.com
Email: info@elivapress.com
Website: www.elivapress.com

This Eliva Press imprint is published by the registered company Eliva Press Global Ltd. part of Eliva Press S.R.L. Publishing Group

The registered company address is: Pope Hennessy Street Level 2, Hennessy Tower Port Louis, Mauritius
Eliva Press S.R.L. Publishing Group legal address is: Bd. Cuza-Voda 1/4 of. 21, Chisinau, Moldova, Europe

SILENT STORM

Inside the World of Asthma

What No One Tells You About Living, Breathing, and Thriving with the World's Most Common Lung Disease

Introduction: The Storm Nobody Sees

It arrives without warning. One moment you are standing in a field, laughing, walking, living — and then, as though a hand has reached inside your chest and closed a fist around your lungs, everything changes. The air that was abundant a second ago is suddenly scarce, precious, rationed. The world contracts to a single, urgent negotiation: the next breath.

Asthma is called a silent storm because its most dangerous moments are often invisible to the people watching from the outside. A person having an asthma attack looks distressed but not obviously broken. There is no blood, no fracture, no dramatic sign visible to bystanders. And yet, inside — in the branching network of airways that supplies life-giving oxygen to every cell in the body — a catastrophic physiological drama is unfolding.

This book tells the full story of that drama: its science, its history, its human faces, and — most importantly — the extraordinary toolkit of knowledge and treatments that can quiet the storm for most of the 300 million people living with asthma today.

Silent Storm is written for the patient who wants to understand their condition at a deeper level than a ten-minute consultation allows. For the parent who lies awake listening to a child's breathing. For the teacher, coach, or colleague who wants to know what to do when someone in their care cannot breathe. And for the curious mind that simply wants to understand one of the most fascinating, complex, and consequential diseases in human history.

The science within these pages reflects the current consensus of international asthma guidelines and peer-reviewed research. The language aims for clarity without sacrificing accuracy. And the spirit of the book is one of honest optimism: asthma is serious, but it is manageable. The storm can be quieted.

✦ PART 1 ✦

Storm Warning

Understanding Asthma

The word 'asthma' comes from the ancient Greek ἆσθμα — asthma — meaning panting or short-drawn breath. It appears in the writings of Hippocrates in the 5th century BCE. It was described by Chinese physicians 2,500 years ago. It has been documented in virtually every human civilization in recorded history.

And yet, despite this long acquaintance with the disease, asthma remains one of the most misunderstood, mismanaged, and underestimated conditions in modern medicine. People with asthma are told their condition is 'just' asthma. They are given inhalers and sent home with minimal education. They are expected to manage a complex, variable, potentially fatal chronic disease with instructions that would not be adequate for operating a coffee machine.

This book begins by establishing the truth about asthma: what it actually is, how widely it affects humanity, and why it demands the respect — from patients, families, and healthcare systems — that so far it has rarely received.

Asthma: A Definition That Does Justice to Complexity

Asthma is a chronic inflammatory disease of the lower respiratory airways characterised by: variable and reversible airflow obstruction; airway hyperresponsiveness to a wide range of stimuli; and underlying airway inflammation that persists even in the absence of symptoms. It is episodic in its manifestation but permanent in its underlying biology — the inflammatory terrain is always present, even when the patient feels well.

This definition immediately reveals why 'just asthma' is such a dangerous phrase. The inflammation is never fully absent. The hyperresponsiveness is always lurking. The potential for a life-threatening episode exists at all times. Asthma is not a condition that comes and goes — only its symptoms do.

The Staggering Global Burden

📊 The Global Footprint of Asthma

339 million people currently diagnosed worldwide (WHO, 2024)
Asthma is the most common chronic disease in children globally
~250,000 deaths per year — 99% in low- and middle-income countries
Asthma rates have increased 50% per decade in high-income countries since the 1960s
Cost to the US economy alone: exceeds $80 billion annually
In Indonesia, asthma affects approximately 11–12% of the population — over 30 million people
Up to 60% of patients have uncontrolled asthma despite having access to medication

Types and Subtypes: The Asthma Family

Modern asthma science recognises that the word 'asthma' covers a family of related but distinct conditions — each with a somewhat different biology, trigger profile, and optimal treatment strategy. The key division is between Type 2-high asthma (driven by eosinophilic and allergic inflammation — the most common form) and Type 2-low asthma (driven by neutrophilic or other mechanisms, often linked to obesity, smoking, or occupational exposure).

Asthma Subtype	Key Characteristics
Allergic (Atopic)	Most common; IgE-mediated; triggered by allergens; begins in childhood; high FeNO
Non-Allergic	No allergic sensitisation; often adult-onset; irritant-triggered; lower FeNO
Exercise-Induced	EIB in up to 90% of asthmatics; cold/dry air triggers; highly treatable
Occupational	Caused/worsened by workplace exposures; affects 10–15% of adult asthma
Aspirin-Exacerbated	NSAID/aspirin triggers; often with nasal polyps; COX-1 pathway
Severe Refractory	5–10% of patients; uncontrolled despite maximal therapy; candidate for biologics
Cough-Variant	Chronic cough as the sole/dominant symptom; frequently misdiagnosed

The Control Imperative

The central clinical goal in asthma is not cure — we do not yet have one — but control. Controlled asthma means: no daytime symptoms; no nocturnal awakening; no limitation of activities; no need for rescue medication (or need fewer than twice weekly); normal or near-normal lung function; and no severe exacerbations.

This level of control is achievable in the vast majority of patients with currently available treatment. The fact that most patients do not achieve it is one of the great unresolved challenges of respiratory medicine.

"Asthma control is not a distant dream — it is a realistic daily reality for anyone who has the right knowledge, the right treatment, and the right support."

✦ PART 2 ✦

The Architecture of Breath

Airway Biology in Health and Disease

To understand why asthma causes such suffering, and why its treatments work the way they do, we need to take a journey through the respiratory system — from the nose to the alveoli, and into the microscopic world of the airway wall where the real action of asthma takes place.

The Respiratory Tree: Form Follows Function

The lungs contain approximately 300 million alveoli — tiny, bubble-like structures with walls so thin that gases can pass freely between the airspace and the adjacent capillary blood. To supply all these alveoli with air, the lung has evolved an elegant branching architecture: the trachea divides into two mainstem bronchi, which divide into lobar and segmental bronchi, which divide into increasingly smaller bronchioles, which finally terminate in the alveolar ducts and alveolar sacs.

The total surface area of the alveolar membrane in a healthy adult is approximately 70 square metres — the size of a singles tennis court — contained within a chest volume of roughly 6 litres. This extraordinary feat of biological engineering supports the gas exchange that sustains every function of the human body.

The Airway Wall: Five Layers of Complexity

The airway wall is not a simple tube — it is a multi-layered biological structure, each layer playing a specific role in normal airway function and each layer altered in characteristic ways by asthma.

Layer	Normal Function	Asthma Changes
Epithelium	Barrier, mucus secretion, cilia-driven clearance	Damaged, leaky; goblet cell hyperplasia; vulnerability to viruses
Basement Membrane	Structural support; filtration	Thickened by collagen deposition (remodeling)

Submucosa	Houses glands, nerves, vessels	Oedema; inflammatory cell infiltration; gland hypertrophy
Smooth Muscle	Regulates airway calibre	Hypertrophy and hyperplasia; exaggerated contraction
Adventitia	Outer support layer	Increased vascularity; neovascularisation

The Inflammatory Cascade: How an Attack Unfolds

An asthma attack is the clinical expression of a well-defined immunological cascade. When a trigger — allergen, virus, cold air, irritant — contacts the sensitised asthmatic airway, it initiates a sequence of events involving dozens of cell types and hundreds of molecular signals. The result, within minutes, is the triad of bronchoconstriction, mucosal oedema, and mucus hypersecretion that defines an acute episode.

Step 1 — Trigger Recognition

Dendritic cells and mast cells stationed throughout the airway epithelium detect the incoming trigger. In allergic asthma, this detection is mediated by IgE antibodies previously produced during sensitisation to that specific allergen. The binding of allergen to IgE on mast cell surfaces is the critical 'recognition event' that initiates the cascade.

Step 2 — Immediate Mediator Release

Within seconds of trigger recognition, mast cells degranulate — releasing preformed mediators including histamine, prostaglandins, and leukotrienes. These molecules act on airway smooth muscle (causing contraction), blood vessels (causing dilation and leakiness), and sensory nerves (causing cough and the sensation of breathlessness). This immediate response explains why symptoms begin within minutes of allergen exposure.

Step 3 — Late-Phase Amplification

Hours later, a second inflammatory wave — the late-phase response — is orchestrated by Th2 lymphocytes releasing IL-4, IL-5, and IL-13. These cytokines recruit eosinophils into the airway, further amplify mucus production, and sustain the inflammatory milieu that keeps the airway hyperresponsive for days after the initial trigger is gone.

Step 4 — Resolution (or Progression to Chronicity)

In mild attacks, the inflammatory cascade resolves. In poorly managed, frequently recurring asthma, each cycle of inflammation and incomplete resolution adds another layer of structural change to the airway wall — the process of remodeling. Scar tissue replaces normal epithelium. Smooth muscle becomes permanently thicker. Airways become irreversibly narrowed.

> **Why Remodeling Matters: The 10-Year Warning**
>
> Research shows that asthma patients with poor long-term control lose lung function at approximately 3x the rate of the general population.
>
> By the time many adults with longstanding asthma are in their 50s and 60s, their airways show features indistinguishable from COPD.
>
> This accelerated lung function decline is largely preventable with consistent inhaled corticosteroid therapy started early.
>
> Every year of inadequate asthma control is a year of lung function being traded away. The debt cannot be repaid.

✦ PART 3 ✦

What Lights the Match

Triggers and Provocation

A trigger is not the cause of asthma — it is the spark that ignites a fire already laid. The kindling is the underlying inflammation and airway hyperresponsiveness; the trigger is simply the agent that sets it off. Understanding your triggers is the most practical, immediately empowering knowledge you can bring to your asthma self-management.

The Major Trigger Categories

1. Aeroallergens — The Invisible Cloud

Aeroallergens are airborne particles of biological origin capable of provoking IgE-mediated allergic responses in sensitised individuals. They are pervasive — impossible to avoid entirely — but their concentration in the immediate environment can be substantially reduced with appropriate measures.

- House dust mites (HDM): The most important indoor allergen globally. Thrive in bedding, carpets, and soft furnishings at temperatures 20–25°C and humidity > 50%. The allergenic proteins are contained in their excreta — tiny enough (1–10 μm diameter) to penetrate to the smallest airways.
- Cockroach allergen: Especially important in urban, low-income environments. Allergens are present in body parts, saliva, and feces. Control requires professional extermination combined with thorough hygiene measures.
- Pet allergens: Cat (Fel d 1) and dog (Can f 1) allergens are extraordinarily sticky and persistent — detectable in cat-free homes for months after a cat has been removed, and commonly transported on clothing into schools and offices.
- Mold spores: Both indoor (Alternaria, Aspergillus, Cladosporium) and outdoor (Alternaria, Cladosporium) molds release spores that can trigger severe asthma. Alternaria is specifically associated with sudden-onset, severe, potentially fatal asthma attacks in young people.
- Seasonal pollens: Tree pollens (spring), grass pollens (late spring/summer), weed pollens (autumn). Climate change is significantly extending pollen seasons and increasing average pollen concentrations across the Northern Hemisphere.

2. Respiratory Viruses — The Most Common Trigger

Rhinovirus — the common cold — is responsible for the majority of asthma exacerbations in both children and adults, causing 60–80% of asthma attacks in school-age children. The virus directly infects airway epithelial cells, amplifying the existing inflammatory milieu and dramatically increasing airway hyperresponsiveness. The resulting exacerbation can persist for weeks after the acute infection has resolved.

COVID-19 has emerged as a clinically important asthma trigger, with SARS-CoV-2 infection causing more severe and prolonged asthma exacerbations than typical rhinovirus infections in many patients. Annual influenza vaccination is strongly recommended for all people with asthma.

3. Air Pollution — The Environmental Emergency

The relationship between air quality and asthma is not subtle — it is profound, well-documented, and worsening as climate change drives higher temperatures, more wildfires, and more extreme weather patterns. Ground-level ozone, fine particulate matter (PM2.5), nitrogen dioxide, and sulfur dioxide all independently worsen asthma and increase the risk of emergency department visits and hospitalisation.

The indoor environment is often overlooked but equally important. Gas cooking stoves produce nitrogen dioxide concentrations that can exceed WHO outdoor air quality guidelines even in well-ventilated kitchens. Scented candles, air fresheners, and many household cleaning products release volatile organic compounds (VOCs) that are potent airway irritants in sensitive individuals.

4. Exercise — The Trigger That Should Not Be Avoided

Exercise-induced bronchoconstriction (EIB) affects up to 90% of people with asthma. The mechanism is primarily osmotic: rapid breathing dries the airway lining, increasing the osmolarity of the airway surface liquid, which triggers mast cell mediator release. Cold, dry air — as encountered during outdoor winter exercise — is the most potent physical trigger.

> **Exercise and Asthma: Strategies for Athletes**
>
> Pre-treatment protocol: SABA (salbutamol 200mcg) via pMDI+spacer 15 minutes before exercise — highly effective in > 80% of EIB.

Warm-up: A 10-minute gradual warm-up at 50–60% max heart rate can 'exhaust' the EIB response, reducing symptoms during the main exercise session.
Nasal breathing: Trains during low-intensity phases; nasal passages warm and humidify air more effectively than the mouth.
Montelukast: Leukotriene receptor antagonist taken daily is effective for exercise-induced symptoms not controlled by pre-treatment alone.
Swimming: Warm, humid pool air is the most EIB-friendly environment; water sports have lower EIB rates than field sports.
Reminder: Olympic-level athletes compete with asthma. With proper management, EIB is rarely a barrier to elite performance.

5. Medications That Trigger Asthma

Several medication classes are well-established asthma triggers and must be used with extreme caution — or avoided entirely — in asthmatic patients.

Drug Class	Risk and Mechanism
NSAIDs (aspirin, ibuprofen, diclofenac)	10–20% of adult asthmatics; COX-1 inhibition diverts arachidonic acid to leukotriene pathway; can cause severe, rapid bronchospasm
Non-selective beta-blockers	Directly block beta-2 receptors; can cause fatal bronchospasm; even eye drops penetrate systemically
ACE inhibitors	Cough (dry) in 10–20% of users; can exacerbate or mimic asthma; switch to ARB if needed
Sulfite preservatives	Found in wine, dried fruit, processed foods; trigger reactions in sulfite-sensitive asthmatics

✦ PART 4 ✦

Reading the Storm

Symptoms, Patterns & Emergency Recognition

Asthma speaks — but its language must be learned. Its symptoms are real and measurable, but they can be mimicked by other conditions, masked by adaptation, or dismissed by those who have not been taught to recognise them. This chapter teaches you to read the storm: to understand what symptoms mean, to recognise dangerous patterns, and to know with absolute certainty when an emergency is unfolding.

The Cardinal Symptoms

Four symptoms define the clinical picture of asthma. In most patients, some combination of these four is present — though the weighting between them varies enormously.

Asthma's Four Cardinal Symptoms

1. WHEEZE — A musical, high-pitched sound during breathing, especially on exhalation. Caused by turbulent airflow through narrowed airways. Not all asthma wheezes; absence of wheeze does not rule out the diagnosis.
2. DYSPNOEA — Shortness of breath; the sensation of air hunger or breathing requiring excessive effort. In asthma, often described as inability to breathe out fully, or a tightness preventing a full breath in.
3. CHEST TIGHTNESS — A sensation of pressure, constriction, or heaviness across the sternum. May precede other symptoms by hours. Frequently misattributed to cardiac causes.
4. COUGH — Typically dry, nonproductive, worse at night and early morning. May be the sole symptom (cough-variant asthma). Often persists after other symptoms have resolved.

The Nocturnal Signature

If there is one pattern that most reliably distinguishes asthma from other causes of respiratory symptoms, it is nocturnal worsening. Asthma symptoms — particularly cough and chest tightness — follow a predictable circadian rhythm, reaching their nadir of airway calibre and peak of symptoms in the early hours of the morning (typically 2–5 a.m.).

This nocturnal predilection reflects several converging physiological processes: the natural trough of endogenous cortisol (which has anti-inflammatory properties); heightened cholinergic airway tone during sleep; cooling of the airways in cooler nighttime air; and horizontal posture increasing airway secretions and reducing functional residual capacity.

Any patient reporting nighttime awakening due to respiratory symptoms — however infrequently — has asthma that is NOT well controlled. This is not a minor inconvenience; it is a clinical signal requiring treatment adjustment.

Prodromal Symptoms: The Storm's Advance Warning

Many experienced asthma patients learn to recognise subtle pre-attack warning signs that appear hours before the classic symptoms develop. These prodromal signals are highly individual but may include: unusual fatigue or mood change; mild rhinorrhoea or sneezing; a tickling or itching sensation at the back of the throat; skin pallor; or vague anxiety without obvious cause.

Recognising and responding to prodromal symptoms — by initiating the yellow-zone response in the action plan — is one of the most effective ways to prevent a mild episode from escalating to a severe one.

Grading the Storm: Mild to Life-Threatening

Feature	Moderate Attack	Severe / Life-Threatening
Speech	Short phrases	Single words or mute
Position	Prefers to sit up	Cannot lie down; tripod posture
Breathing rate	20–30/min	> 30/min or paradoxically slow
Wheeze	Moderate	Loud OR SILENT (very dangerous)
SABA response	Partial	None
Oxygen saturation	91–95%	< 91%; cyanosis
Action required	Contact doctor urgently	Call emergency services NOW

🚨 The Silent Chest — The Most Dangerous Sign in Asthma

A chest that makes no wheeze during a severe asthma attack is not an improvement — it is a medical emergency.

Silence occurs when airways are so severely narrowed that insufficient air is moving to produce turbulent sound.

This is a sign of imminent respiratory failure.

Call emergency services (119 in Indonesia / 000 in Australia / 911 in the US) IMMEDIATELY.

Administer oxygen if available. Do NOT wait to see if it improves.

✦ PART 5 ✦

Pinning Down the Storm

Diagnosis — Tests That Tell the Truth

A diagnosis of asthma should be both clinically suspected AND objectively confirmed. In practice, asthma is frequently over-diagnosed (other conditions labelled as asthma without proper testing) and under-diagnosed (genuine asthma attributed to other causes for years). Both errors carry serious consequences. This chapter explains what a rigorous asthma diagnosis looks like and why it matters.

Why Symptoms Alone Are Not Enough

Wheeze, dyspnoea, chest tightness, and cough are non-specific symptoms that can be caused by dozens of conditions besides asthma. Heart failure causes nocturnal dyspnoea. Vocal cord dysfunction causes episodic wheeze. COPD causes fixed airflow obstruction. Bronchiectasis causes chronic cough. Diagnosing any of these as asthma — and treating them with inhalers — can delay the correct diagnosis for years and expose patients to unnecessary and potentially harmful treatment.

Spirometry: The Non-Negotiable Foundation

Spirometry is the gold standard for confirming the presence and severity of airflow obstruction. It should be performed before any diagnosis of asthma is made in adults and school-age children. Yet surveys consistently show that spirometry is not performed in a substantial minority of new asthma diagnoses — a serious quality gap in asthma care.

What Spirometry Measures and What It Means

FEV1 (Forced Expiratory Volume in 1 second): Volume of air expelled in the first second of maximal effort.
→ Reduced in airflow obstruction. < 80% of predicted value = significant reduction.
FVC (Forced Vital Capacity): Total volume expelled in a maximal forced exhalation.
→ May be reduced in restriction or severe obstruction.
FEV1/FVC ratio: The key obstructive index.
→ < 0.70 (70%) in adults = airflow obstruction present.

Post-bronchodilator reversibility: FEV1 improves ≥ 12% AND ≥ 200ml after SABA inhalation.
→ Positive reversibility is the hallmark of asthma, distinguishing it from fixed obstruction (COPD).
Peak Expiratory Flow (PEF) variability: > 20% diurnal variation over 4 weeks = strongly supports asthma.

FeNO: Seeing the Inflammation

Fractional exhaled nitric oxide (FeNO) is a non-invasive test that measures eosinophilic airway inflammation directly — something that spirometry cannot do. The patient breathes out at a controlled flow rate through a handheld analyser that calculates the nitric oxide concentration in exhaled air within 10 seconds.

- FeNO > 50 ppb: High probability of eosinophilic (Type 2) inflammation; strong predictor of ICS response.
- FeNO 25–50 ppb: Intermediate; interpret in clinical context.
- FeNO < 25 ppb: Low probability of eosinophilic inflammation; consider non-Type 2 asthma or alternative diagnosis.

FeNO is particularly useful for monitoring ICS adherence: a patient whose FeNO was previously well-suppressed but has risen at their next appointment has most likely been skipping doses — a finding that can guide an adherence-focused consultation rather than unnecessary medication escalation.

The Diagnostic Workup: A Systematic Approach

1. Detailed clinical history — symptom pattern, triggers, nocturnal symptoms, atopic history, occupational exposures, medication use, smoking history.
2. Physical examination — during an episode: wheeze, hyperinflation, tachypnoea; between episodes: often normal.
3. Spirometry with bronchodilator reversibility test — required for all adults and children > 5 years.
4. FeNO measurement — to characterise inflammatory phenotype.
5. Skin prick tests or specific IgE — to identify allergen sensitisation.
6. If spirometry normal: bronchial challenge testing (methacholine PC20) and/or peak flow diary.

7. Blood eosinophil count — to characterise inflammatory phenotype for treatment selection.

Conditions That Mimic Asthma

Mimic Condition	Distinguishing Clues
COPD	Age > 40; smoking > 10 pack-years; FEV1/FVC < 0.70 without reversibility; emphysema on CT
Vocal Cord Dysfunction	Inspiratory stridor; normal spirometry between episodes; psychological history
Cardiac Failure	Orthopnoea; ankle oedema; raised BNP; history of cardiac disease; responds to diuretics
Bronchiectasis	Chronic productive cough; recurrent infections; CT shows dilated thick-walled airways
Tracheal Stenosis	Fixed monophonic wheeze over trachea; flow-volume loop shows fixed obstruction
Hyperventilation	Tingling, dizziness; low CO2; responds to breathing retraining; normal spirometry

✦ PART 6 ✦

The Pharmacopoeia

Medications for Asthma Explained

Modern asthma pharmacology offers a therapeutic range that stretches from simple, inexpensive inhalers available in any pharmacy to highly sophisticated biological agents that cost tens of thousands of dollars per year and target single molecular pathways with extraordinary precision. Understanding this spectrum — what each drug does, why it works, and when it is appropriate — transforms a patient from a passive recipient of prescriptions into an active partner in their own care.

The Preventer vs. Reliever Divide

The single most important concept in asthma pharmacology is the distinction between medications that prevent attacks and medications that relieve them. These are not interchangeable. They work by entirely different mechanisms, on different timescales, and they address different aspects of the disease.

PREVENTERS	RELIEVERS
Work over days to weeks	Work within 2–5 minutes
Target airway inflammation	Target airway smooth muscle (bronchoconstriction)
Must be taken DAILY regardless of symptoms	Taken ONLY when symptoms occur (or before exercise)
Examples: ICS, ICS/LABA, LTRA, biologics	Examples: salbutamol, terbutaline, formoterol (in MART)
Address the fire	Open a window during the fire
Taking alone without preventer = dangerous	Overuse (> 2x/week) = sign of poor control

Inhaled Corticosteroids — The Cornerstone

Inhaled corticosteroids — budesonide, fluticasone propionate, fluticasone furoate, beclomethasone dipropionate, ciclesonide, mometasone — have been the most transformative medication class in asthma management since their introduction in the 1970s. Their mechanism is complex: they suppress the transcription of multiple pro-inflammatory genes within airway epithelial and immune cells, reducing eosinophil recruitment, decreasing mucus gland secretion, and restoring epithelial barrier function.

The evidence base for ICS is among the most robust in all of clinical medicine: dozens of large randomised controlled trials consistently show 50% reductions in severe exacerbations, 50% reductions in asthma hospitalisations, and approximately 50% reduction in asthma mortality compared with bronchodilator-only treatment.

> ⭐ ICS Safety: What the Evidence Actually Shows
>
> LOW-MEDIUM DOSE ICS (the dose used by most patients): Extremely safe. Systemic absorption is negligible.
> LOCAL SIDE EFFECTS: Oral thrush (candidiasis) and dysphonia (hoarse voice) occur in ~5% — prevented by rinsing mouth after use and using a spacer.
> HIGH DOSE ICS: Some evidence of mild bone density reduction, mild skin thinning at very high long-term doses.
> CHILDREN'S HEIGHT: Slight reduction in growth velocity at high doses; does NOT affect final adult height; uncontrolled asthma itself impairs growth more.
> BOTTOM LINE: No patient with persistent asthma should be denied ICS because of fear of steroid side effects. The risk/benefit balance is overwhelmingly favourable.

Combination Inhalers: ICS + LABA

When asthma is not controlled on moderate-dose ICS alone, adding a long-acting beta-2 agonist (LABA) to the ICS produces superior outcomes to simply increasing the ICS dose. LABAs — salmeterol, formoterol, vilanterol, indacaterol — provide 12–24 hours of bronchodilation, complementing the anti-inflammatory effect of ICS.

Fixed-dose combination inhalers (ICS + LABA in a single device) have largely replaced separate inhalers in current practice because they guarantee that the two drugs are always taken together — preventing the dangerous scenario of a patient taking LABA without ICS.

The MART Strategy: A Paradigm Shift

Maintenance And Reliever Therapy (MART) uses a single ICS/formoterol inhaler for both daily maintenance dosing AND as-needed symptom relief. Because formoterol has a rapid onset (comparable to salbutamol) combined with an 8–12 hour duration, it can serve both purposes. Every time a patient takes an extra rescue puff during symptoms, they automatically receive an additional dose of ICS — providing anti-inflammatory coverage precisely when inflammation is peaking.

Multiple large trials — including the landmark SYGMA studies — have shown MART to be superior to separate preventer + reliever regimens in reducing severe exacerbations, and inferior to fixed high-dose maintenance only for the most severe patients. Current GINA guidelines recommend MART as the preferred strategy for Steps 3–5.

Biologic Therapies: Precision Targeting

Biologic monoclonal antibodies represent the most significant advance in severe asthma treatment of the past two decades. By targeting individual cytokines or receptors in the asthmatic inflammatory cascade, they can dramatically reduce attacks, eliminate the need for chronic oral steroids, and improve quality of life in patients whose disease was previously uncontrollable.

Biologic (Brand)	Primary Target and Indication
Omalizumab (Xolair)	Anti-IgE; allergic asthma with elevated total IgE; reduces mast cell activation
Mepolizumab (Nucala)	Anti-IL-5; severe eosinophilic asthma (blood eos ≥ 150–300 cells/μL)
Benralizumab (Fasenra)	Anti-IL-5Rα; rapid complete eosinophil depletion; every 8 weeks after loading
Dupilumab (Dupixent)	Anti-IL-4Rα; blocks IL-4 and IL-13; effective in Type 2 asthma + eczema + CRS
Tezepelumab (Tezspire)	Anti-TSLP; broadest action; effective regardless of eosinophil count or IgE

Biologics are not appropriate for all asthma patients — they are reserved for severe, uncontrolled disease (typically Step 4–5) in patients who meet specific biomarker criteria. But for those patients, they can be genuinely life-changing: 50–70% reductions in exacerbation rates, dramatic reductions in oral steroid dependency, and restoration of normal daily function.

✦ PART 7 ✦

The Delivery Problem

Inhalers, Devices, and the Art of Getting Medication to the Lungs

Here is an uncomfortable truth: even the most effective asthma medication in the world is useless if it never reaches the part of the lung where it is needed. And the research tells us that, for most patients, it does not — because inhaler technique is almost universally poor.

Studies conducted across multiple countries and healthcare settings consistently find that 70–80% of patients make at least one critical error in their inhaler technique. These errors reduce the proportion of medication reaching the lungs by 50–80%. The practical consequence: patients appear to be on adequate treatment but are receiving a fraction of the prescribed dose.

Why Inhaler Technique Matters So Much

Inhaled medication faces a formidable delivery challenge. The target — the small airways where asthmatic inflammation is most intense — is deep within the lung, accessible only to particles small enough to avoid impacting on the back of the throat, the trachea, or the larger bronchi. For medication to reach the target:

- Particles must be in the respirable range (1–5 μm diameter).
- They must be delivered at an appropriate velocity and flow rate.
- The patient must generate adequate inspiratory flow (for DPIs) or coordinate actuation with inspiration (for pMDIs).
- The breath must be held long enough for particles to settle by sedimentation.

Every inhaler device has a specific technique that optimises these conditions. Deviation from correct technique at any step reduces lung deposition and wastes medication.

Pressurised Metered-Dose Inhaler (pMDI)

The classic 'puffer' has been the dominant inhaler device for 60 years. It uses a chemical propellant (now HFA, replacing the ozone-depleting CFC of earlier generations) to aerosolise a precisely measured dose. The challenge is that the aerosol is released at high velocity — approximately 100 km/h — and patients who breathe in too fast or press the canister at the wrong moment will deposit most of the dose in the back of their throat.

▮ pMDI Masterclass — Common Errors and Corrections

ERROR: Pressing the canister BEFORE starting to breathe in.
→ CORRECTION: Start inhaling slowly first, then press while continuing the slow, deep breath.
ERROR: Breathing in too FAST — a sharp, forceful inhalation.
→ CORRECTION: Inhale as slowly and deeply as possible over 3–5 seconds.
ERROR: Not holding the breath afterwards.
→ CORRECTION: Hold for 10 seconds (or as long as comfortable) to allow deposition.
ERROR: Actuation without shaking the inhaler first.
→ CORRECTION: Shake vigorously for 5 seconds before every use.
ERROR: Multiple actuations with a single breath.
→ CORRECTION: One actuation per breath; wait 30–60 seconds between doses.

Spacers and Holding Chambers

A spacer eliminates the coordination problem entirely. The aerosol from the pMDI is released into the spacer chamber, where it slows, the propellant evaporates, and the particle size optimises — after which the patient inhales at their own pace. Lung deposition increases from ~15–20% (pMDI alone) to ~30–40% (pMDI + spacer). Throat deposition — and therefore oral candidiasis risk with ICS — decreases dramatically.

Every patient using a pMDI for maintenance ICS therapy should be using a spacer. Children below school age should use a spacer with a face mask. During acute asthma attacks, a pMDI + spacer is as effective as a nebuliser for bronchodilator delivery — and significantly faster to prepare.

Dry Powder Inhalers (DPIs)

DPIs use the patient's own inspiratory effort to disperse the medication. They are breath-actuated — no coordination of hand and breath is required — but they do require a minimum inspiratory flow (typically 30–60 L/min depending on the device). This requirement makes DPIs less suitable for young children, severely breathless patients, and those with significantly reduced inspiratory capacity.

Each DPI device has a specific loading mechanism and inhalation profile. The Turbuhaler, Accuhaler, Ellipta, Handihaler, and Breezhaler all work differently. A patient switching from one DPI to another — even for the same drug — needs specific retraining for the new device.

Smart Inhalers – The Digital Revolution

Electronic adherence monitoring sensors that attach to conventional inhalers — or are incorporated into new device designs — are transforming the ability to measure and improve inhaler use in real-world settings. These devices record every actuation with timestamp, detect errors in technique (insufficient shake, inadequate flow), measure ambient temperature and humidity, and sync data to smartphone apps.

The Propeller Health system, Adherium Smartinhaler, and several built-in smart inhaler designs have demonstrated in clinical trials that real-time adherence monitoring and feedback reduce asthma attacks, reduce emergency department visits, and improve asthma control scores compared with conventional care. Several health systems are now implementing smart inhaler programmes as standard of care for difficult-to-control asthma.

✦ PART 8 ✦

A Lifetime Storm

Asthma at Every Age

Asthma is not a fixed experience. It changes with development, adapts to hormones, responds to life circumstances, and presents entirely different challenges at 3 years, 13 years, 33 years, and 63 years. The person who manages their asthma well is the one who understands not just the condition in general but their relationship with it at the particular life stage they occupy.

Before School: The Wheezing Infant

Infant and toddler wheeze presents a diagnostic and management challenge that is unique in asthma medicine. Up to one-third of children wheeze during at least one of their first three years of life — but fewer than half of these will go on to have persistent asthma. Transient early wheeze (caused by small airways, not inflammation) can be clinically indistinguishable from early atopic asthma.

Predictors of persistent asthma in wheezy infants include: parental asthma or eczema; the infant having eczema themselves; blood eosinophilia; positive specific IgE to common allergens; and wheeze that occurs in the absence of respiratory infections. These 'API' (Asthma Predictive Index) criteria help clinicians identify infants at highest risk and most likely to benefit from early preventive therapy.

School Age: The Social Dimension

Asthma is the leading cause of school absence due to chronic disease. It affects physical education participation, social interaction, sleep quality, and cognitive performance (through nocturnal symptoms and medication side effects). Children with asthma are at elevated risk of anxiety, bullying, and reduced self-esteem — particularly if their condition is not well understood by school staff and peers.

School and Asthma: A Checklist

✓ Provide the school with a written, signed Asthma Action Plan before the academic year begins.
✓ Ensure both the school nurse/office AND the child's bag contain a rescue inhaler.
✓ Brief the child's class teacher on early warning signs of an attack.
✓ Pre-treatment with SABA before physical education — arrange with the PE teacher.
✓ Discuss asthma openly with your child in age-appropriate language — shame is dangerous.
✓ Address triggers in the school environment: mold, chalk dust, outdoor pollen exposure.
✓ Attendance at regular asthma review is as important as school attendance itself.

Adolescence: The Perfect Storm

No life stage combines higher intrinsic asthma risk with greater barriers to management than adolescence. Teenagers are simultaneously: at a biological age when asthma severity and hyperresponsiveness may be increasing; likely to be experimenting with tobacco, cannabis, and alcohol (all airway irritants or inflammatory stimulants); motivated to conceal their condition to avoid social stigma; and developmentally programmed to underestimate personal risk.

Asthma fatality rates in teenagers are disproportionate to the severity of their disease — driven primarily by delayed action, poor adherence, and overconfidence during attacks. Studies of fatal asthma in young people consistently find the same patterns: heavy SABA use without preventer therapy; failure to seek emergency help despite prolonged severe symptoms; and social isolation during the attack (alone in a room, late at night).

Talking to Teenagers About Asthma Risk

Emphasise capability and control, not limitation — framing asthma as 'manageable' resonates more than framing it as 'dangerous'.
Be explicit about the specific risks: 'not taking your preventer doubles your risk of a serious attack'.
Discuss drugs and alcohol honestly — cannabis is a powerful airway irritant; alcohol can trigger attacks.
Involve teenagers in creating their own action plan — ownership improves adherence.
Ensure the teenager knows what a severe attack looks and feels like, and has a clear instruction to call for help.

Pregnancy and Asthma

Asthma affects 4–12% of pregnant women, making it the most common chronic medical condition requiring treatment during pregnancy. The key clinical message — that all approved asthma medications are safer than uncontrolled asthma for the developing baby — cannot be overstated.

Uncontrolled asthma in pregnancy is associated with preterm birth, intrauterine growth restriction, neonatal hypoxia, and perinatal mortality. These outcomes are caused by the direct effect of maternal hypoxia on fetal oxygen supply during asthma attacks. Well-controlled asthma, by contrast, carries no significant additional obstetric risk above the general population.

Older Adults and Late-Onset Asthma

Adult-onset asthma (first diagnosed in adults) is more common than generally recognised and tends to be non-allergic, more persistent, and less responsive to standard therapy than childhood-onset asthma. It is frequently associated with obesity, smoking, occupational exposures, female sex hormones (increasing incidence around menopause), and aspirin sensitivity.

In patients over 65, asthma is under-diagnosed (often attributed to COPD, cardiac failure, or 'getting older'), and inhaler technique is frequently poor due to arthritis, reduced grip strength, and cognitive factors. Comorbidities — cardiac disease requiring beta-blockers, musculoskeletal disease requiring NSAIDs — can directly worsen asthma or complicate its management.

✦ PART 9 ✦

Storm Management

Your Daily Action System

The difference between surviving with asthma and thriving with it comes down, in most cases, to a system. Not willpower. Not luck. Not severity. A system: a consistent set of daily habits, monitoring tools, environmental adaptations, and pre-planned responses that keep the storm from building and give you a clear path when it begins to.

Component 1: Your Written Asthma Action Plan

The written Asthma Action Plan (AAP) is the single most evidence-based intervention in asthma self-management. Patients with written AAPs have 50% fewer hospitalisations and significantly fewer emergency department visits than those without. And yet, fewer than 30% of people with asthma have one.

A complete AAP contains five elements:

8. Your daily medications — names, doses, frequency, device.
9. Your personal 'Green Zone' definition — what well-controlled asthma feels like for you (by symptoms and/or peak flow).
10. Your 'Yellow Zone' response — how to recognise worsening and what to do (add rescue puffs, increase preventer, contact doctor within X hours).
11. Your 'Red Zone' response — severe symptoms requiring emergency action; exact steps to take before emergency services arrive.
12. Emergency contacts — your doctor's number, the local emergency number, a trusted family member or friend.

Component 2: Peak Flow Monitoring

A peak flow meter costs the price of a modest restaurant meal and can be one of the most powerful tools in asthma self-management. By measuring peak expiratory flow rate daily — ideally morning and evening — you build a personal baseline and can detect significant drops in lung function before symptoms become severe.

Your personal best peak flow (established during a period of excellent control) serves as the 100% reference value. When your morning peak flow drops to 80% of personal best, you are entering the Yellow Zone. When it drops below 60%, you are in the Red Zone and need urgent medical attention — regardless of how you feel subjectively.

> ✓ **Using Peak Flow Effectively**
> Measure at the same times each day (morning and evening are ideal).
> Take the best of 3 attempts — record it in a diary or app.
> Record it BEFORE taking your morning reliever (for a true baseline).
> Diurnal variation > 20% between morning and evening readings = poorly controlled asthma.
> A downward trend over several days is more important than any single reading.
> Share your peak flow diary with your doctor at every review appointment.

Component 3: Environmental Control

Trigger avoidance is unglamorous, effortful, and enormously effective. A 10% reduction in your two most important triggers typically translates into a meaningful reduction in attack frequency. The following environmental modifications are evidence-based and achievable without major expense for most patients.

For dust mite allergy (the most important indoor intervention):

- Allergen-impermeable encasings on mattress, pillow, and duvet — the single most effective dust mite measure.
- Weekly hot wash (≥ 60°C) of all bedding.
- Hard flooring in the bedroom; remove curtains (replace with blinds that can be wiped clean).
- Keep bedroom humidity below 50% using ventilation or a dehumidifier.
- Minimise soft toys; wash any regularly at ≥ 60°C or freeze overnight.

For tobacco smoke (the most important irritant):

- Absolute no-smoking rule inside the home and in the car.

- If the patient smokes: pharmacotherapy (varenicline, NRT) combined with behavioural support is highly effective.
- Passive smoking exposure at any level worsens asthma control and accelerates lung function decline.

Component 4: Adherence Engineering

Adherence to preventer medication is the single most modifiable determinant of asthma outcomes — and the most commonly neglected. Research shows that patients who take their ICS as prescribed have dramatically better outcomes than those who take it intermittently. The challenge is that taking medication when you feel well, for an illness that is not bothering you at that moment, requires a kind of motivated discipline that most human beings find difficult without support structures.

Practical Adherence Strategies That Work

Habit stacking: attach inhaler use to a non-negotiable daily habit — toothbrushing is the most effective anchor (keep inhaler next to toothbrush).

Phone alarms: set a morning and evening alarm labelled with the reason, not just 'medicine' — e.g., 'protect my lungs'.

Dose tracking: use a calendar, a simple tally on paper, or a smartphone app (MyAsthma, AsthmaMD).

Smart inhaler sensors: for patients with persistent poor adherence, electronic monitoring sensors provide objective data and automated reminders.

Understand the 'why': patients who understand that preventers reduce silent airway inflammation — even when feeling well — adhere significantly better than those who see them as 'just in case' medicine.

Address side effect concerns openly with your doctor: they are almost always manageable.

Component 5: Regular Medical Review

Asthma that is well controlled still requires regular review — at least annually, and more frequently during periods of instability. Good asthma care is not a one-time event but an ongoing, dynamic partnership between patient and clinician. A good asthma review should cover: current symptom control (using a validated questionnaire like the Asthma Control Test); inhaler technique observation; peak flow diary review; adherence assessment; update of the written action plan; and discussion of any concerns, side effects, or life changes that might affect asthma management.

✦ PART 10 ✦

After the Storm

The Future of Asthma Care

We are living in the most exciting era in the history of asthma research. The combination of genomics, single-cell transcriptomics, proteomics, digital health, and artificial intelligence is generating insights into asthma's biology at a granularity that was unimaginable even a decade ago. We do not yet have a cure — but we have, for the first time, a credible scientific pathway toward one.

Understanding the Asthma Microbiome

One of the most striking recent findings in asthma research is the profound influence of microbial communities — in the gut, airways, and skin — on the development and severity of asthma. The 'biodiversity hypothesis' proposes that reduced exposure to diverse microbial environments in early childhood (a consequence of urbanisation, antibiotics overuse, caesarean section delivery, and formula feeding) disrupts the normal maturation of immune regulatory pathways, increasing the risk of allergic and asthmatic disease.

Children raised on traditional farms — exposed to a rich diversity of environmental microbes from birth — have dramatically lower rates of asthma and allergy than their urban peers. Researchers are now attempting to identify the specific microbial exposures responsible for this protection, with the goal of developing probiotic or microbial therapy protocols that could replicate the 'farm effect' in urban environments.

Genetics and Epigenetics: Reading the Blueprint

Genome-wide association studies (GWAS) have identified over 100 genetic loci associated with asthma risk — but no single gene determines whether a person develops the condition. Rather, asthma arises from the interaction between multiple genetic variants and environmental exposures across the first years of life.

Perhaps more actionable than the genetic blueprint itself are the epigenetic modifications that alter how genes are expressed — modifications that are influenced by environmental factors and, crucially, may be partially reversible. Research into the epigenetics of asthma is opening potential avenues for therapies that could silence the inflammatory gene expression patterns that drive chronic disease.

Next-Generation Biologics and Small Molecules

The biologic revolution in severe asthma has validated the precision medicine approach — but current biologics address only a subset of inflammatory pathways. The next generation of therapies aims to extend this coverage to more patients and achieve even more complete disease control.

Emerging Therapy	Target and Status
Anti-IL-33 (itepekimab)	Upstream Type 2 alarm signal; Phase 3 trials positive; particularly promising for virus-triggered asthma
Anti-TSLP combinations	Combining tezepelumab with ICS/LABA; investigating synergistic effects
BTK inhibitors (oral)	Small molecule mast cell and B-cell suppression; several in Phase 2/3
JAK inhibitors (inhaled)	Broad anti-cytokine action via inhaled route; potential to replace biologics for some patients
Allergen immunotherapy + biologics	Combining anti-IgE/anti-IL-4 with desensitisation for faster, safer allergen tolerance
mRNA-based tolerance induction	Experimental; aims to induce specific allergen tolerance via mRNA delivery

Artificial Intelligence: Predicting the Storm

Artificial intelligence is beginning to transform asthma medicine in ways that are not merely incremental but genuinely revolutionary. Machine learning algorithms trained on vast datasets of patient-generated data — inhaler use patterns, heart rate variability, sleep quality, GPS location, environmental pollen and pollution data — can predict asthma attacks 24–72 hours before they occur with accuracy that exceeds that of individual clinical assessment.

The Healtheon AI system, developed in collaboration with several UK NHS trusts, demonstrated in a 2023 trial that AI-guided personalised asthma management — using smart inhaler data and environmental inputs — reduced severe exacerbations by 43% compared with standard care. Similar systems are in development by multiple academic medical centres and technology companies worldwide.

The Primary Prevention Horizon

The ultimate goal of asthma research is not better treatment of established disease but prevention of the disease from ever developing. This requires understanding and intervening during the critical developmental window — the first 1,000 days of life — when the immune system, airway architecture, and microbial ecology are being established.

Current prevention research is exploring: maternal and infant probiotic supplementation; vitamin D supplementation during pregnancy and infancy; promotion of breastfeeding; avoidance of unnecessary antibiotic use in infancy; urban green space design that increases microbial biodiversity; and policies to reduce air pollution in the neighborhoods and schools where children spend their early years.

None of these interventions has yet been definitively proven to prevent asthma in large clinical trials — but the biological rationale is strong, the epidemiological evidence is compelling, and several trials are currently underway. The possibility of preventing asthma — rather than simply managing it — is no longer science fiction.

Closing: The Storm That Can Be Quieted

Silent Storm opened with the image of a disease that is invisible from the outside — a physiological drama playing out unseen, unfelt by anyone except the person fighting for air. We close with a different image: the person with asthma who has the knowledge, the tools, and the support to face that storm with confidence.

Asthma is serious. It is chronic. It demands respect and consistent engagement. But it is also, for the vast majority of people who have it, a thoroughly conquerable condition — one that need not define the limits of what is possible in a life.

The 300 million people living with asthma today include Olympic athletes, opera singers, world leaders, scientists, parents, teachers, farmers, and children who will grow up to do extraordinary things. Their asthma is real, but it is not their ceiling.

"It is not the storm that defines you. It is what you do while it is raging."

Quiet the storm. Breathe deeply. Live without limits.

Glossary

Aeroallergen: An airborne allergen capable of provoking respiratory allergic responses, e.g., pollen, dust mite particles, pet dander.

API: Asthma Predictive Index — a scoring tool to estimate the probability that a wheezing infant will develop persistent asthma.

Atopy: The genetic predisposition to develop IgE-mediated allergic diseases including asthma, eczema, and hay fever.

Bronchoconstriction: Narrowing of the airways caused by contraction of airway smooth muscle.

Bronchodilator: A drug that relaxes airway smooth muscle, widening the airways and improving airflow.

Circadian rhythm: The 24-hour biological cycle that influences many physiological processes, including airway inflammation and calibre.

Eosinophil: A type of white blood cell central to Type 2 asthmatic inflammation; elevated in blood or sputum in allergic asthma.

Epigenetics: Modifications to gene expression — not the DNA sequence itself — caused by environmental factors; potentially reversible.

FeNO: Fractional Exhaled Nitric Oxide — a breath test measuring eosinophilic airway inflammation.

FEV1: Forced Expiratory Volume in 1 second — the volume of air expelled in the first second of maximal forced exhalation.

GINA: Global Initiative for Asthma — the international body that publishes evidence-based asthma management guidelines.

ICS: Inhaled Corticosteroid — the cornerstone anti-inflammatory preventer therapy for asthma.

IgE: Immunoglobulin E — the antibody class mediating immediate allergic reactions via mast cells.

LABA: Long-Acting Beta-2 Agonist — bronchodilator with 12–24 hour duration; combined with ICS in persistent asthma.

MART: Maintenance And Reliever Therapy — single ICS/formoterol inhaler for both maintenance and as-needed relief.

Microbiome: The community of microorganisms (bacteria, viruses, fungi) colonising the gut, airways, and skin.

Morbidity: The burden of disease — symptoms, hospitalisations, reduced quality of life.

Peak Flow: Peak Expiratory Flow Rate — the maximum speed of air expelled from the lungs; measured with a peak flow meter.

Remodeling: Irreversible structural changes to the airway wall caused by repeated cycles of inflammation and repair.

SABA: Short-Acting Beta-2 Agonist — rapid-onset bronchodilator (2–5 minutes); used for acute symptom relief.

Spirometry: A lung function test measuring FEV1, FVC, and FEV1/FVC to assess the degree of airflow obstruction.

Type 2 inflammation: The dominant inflammatory pathway in allergic asthma, driven by IL-4, IL-5, IL-13, IgE, and eosinophils.

References and Further Reading

The following sources informed the content of this book and are recommended for further exploration:

- GINA. Global Strategy for Asthma Management and Prevention, 2024. ginasthma.org
- Lambrecht BN & Hammad H. The immunology of asthma. Nature Immunology 2015;16:45–56.
- Brusselle GG et al. New insights into the immunology of chronic obstructive pulmonary disease. Lancet 2011.
- O'Byrne PM et al. Inhaled budesonide-formoterol as needed in mild asthma. NEJM 2018;378:1865–76.
- Menzies-Gow A et al. Tezepelumab in severe, uncontrolled asthma. NEJM 2021;384:1800–09.
- Strachan DP. Hay fever, hygiene, and household size. BMJ 1989 — the original hygiene hypothesis paper.
- Ege MJ et al. Exposure to environmental microorganisms and childhood asthma. NEJM 2011;364:701–09.
- Papi A et al. Budesonide/formoterol as maintenance and reliever therapy in asthma (SYGMA-1). Lancet 2018.
- Reddel HK et al. Heterogeneity within and between physician-diagnosed asthma and/or COPD. Chest 2019.
- WHO. Asthma Fact Sheet. who.int/news-room/fact-sheets/detail/asthma, 2024.
- Asthma and Allergy Foundation of America (AAFA). aafa.org
- Asthma + Lung UK. asthma.org.uk
- National Asthma Council Australia. nationalasthma.org.au

This book is an educational resource and does not constitute medical advice. Individual treatment decisions should always be made in partnership with a qualified healthcare professional.

Publisher: Eliva Press Global Ltd

Email: info@elivapress.com